Please Explain Tonsillectomy & Adenoidectomy to Me

A Complete Guide to Preparing Your Child for Surgery

3rd Edition

By Laurie Zelinger, Ph.D, ABPP, RPT-S and Perry Zelinger, M.D.

D1449891

Loving Healing Press

Ann Arbor, MI

Please Explain Tonsillectomy & Adenoidectomy To Me: A Complete Guide to Preparing Your Child for Surgery, 3rd Edition

Library of Congress Cataloging-in-Publication Data

Names: Zelinger, Laurie E., 1952- author. | Zelinger, Perry, (Perry Joseph) 1991- author.
Title: Please explain tonsillectomy and adenoidectomy to me : a complete guide to preparing your child for surgery / by Laurie Zelinger, Ph.D, R.P.T.-S and Perry Zelinger, M.D.
Other titles: "O, my" in tonsillectomy & adenoidectomy
Description: 3rd edition. | Ann Arbor, MI : Loving Healing Press, [2018] | Revision of: "O, my" in tonsillectomy & adenoidectomy. 2009. | Includes bibliographical references and index.
Identifiers: LCCN 2018043715 (print) | LCCN 2018044323 (ebook) | ISBN 9781615994205 (Kindle, ePub, pdf) | ISBN 9781615994182 (pbk. : alk. paper) | ISBN 9781615994199 (hardcover : alk. paper)
Subjects: LCSH: Tonsillectomy. | Adenoidectomy. | Tonsillitis. | Children--Surgery.
Classification: LCC RF484.5 (ebook) | LCC RF484.5 .Z45 2018 (print) | DDC 617.5/32--dc23
LC record available at https://lccn.loc.gov/2018043715

Published by:
Loving Healing Press
5145 Pontiac Trail
Ann Arbor, MI 48105
USA

http://www.LovingHealing.com or
info@LovingHealing.com
Tollfree 888 761 6268
Fax 734 663 6861

Professionals Praise Please Explain Tonsillectomy & Adenoidectomy to Me

Please Explain Tonsillectomy and Adenoidectomy to Me is a handy and valuable guide for parents who face the ultimate decision to have their child undergo a tonsillectomy or adenoidectomy. So many fear the procedure and procrastinate, but this book unravels the fear, answers the questions and makes it understandable and reassuring. It is much needed in the field and its joyful illustrations make it easy to follow and comprehend. Easy to read and grasp, it is sure to allay most parents' fears and make the surgery clear for both the parent and child. When parents and children are informed, enlightened and understand the process, the child is well positioned to have better health, hearing, speech and language development. It is a winning combination.

Donna Geffner, Ph.D., Ed.D (Hon.), CCC-SP/A
Past President of the American Speech-Language Hearing Association
Honors Recipient, ASHA

Dr. Laurie Zelinger is not only a sought after child psychologist, but also a wonderful author in her own right. It is hard to speak, let alone write, about difficult issues like tonsillectomy to a child. When reading the book, you feel as if Dr. Laurie is right in front of you and leading you through the whole process. This book provides a useful, simple and straight forward approach for parents and children to deal with the anxiety that precedes any surgery.

Zev Ash, M.D., F.A.A.P. (Pediatrician)

As owners and directors of a nursery school and summer camp for the past 27 years, we are often asked how to prepare a child for a medical procedure. Well, who knew preparing for a tonsillectomy meant more than just buying ice cream? This book is an excellent road map for preparing not just the child, but also the parent for a scary and often intimidating experience. It is a soup-to-nuts approach that will help guide you through the unexpected. We wish this book was available when our child had her tonsils removed.

Adam & Amy Langbart,
owners/directors of Merrick Woods Country Day School and Camp, Merrick, NY.

What do parents do when they have just been told that their child needs an invasive medical procedure involving a hospital and anesthesia? Reach for and read, *Please Explain Tonsillectomy and Adenoidectomy to Me*. Blending personal experience, relevant factual references and engaging illustrations, Dr. Laurie Zelinger and Dr. Perry Zelinger present a clear, logical and highly informative book that will guide parents on a journey from the initial visit to the pediatrician to the return home following surgery. The use of actual possible scripts to use with your child to help explain procedures and ease anxiety, well organized helpful to-do lists and timelines serve to make this a required read and practical guide for parents or any caregiver with a child about to undergo a tonsillectomy and adenoidectomy.

Steven H. Blaustein Ph.D, CCC, BCS-CL, Speech-Language Pathologist
Board Certified Specialist- Child Language, Associate Professor- Touro College Graduate
Program, Speech-Language Pathology

Wow! What an amazing book for parents and children. I only wish such a book had been available to me and my parents in 1948, when at age 4, I had a tonsillectomy and suffered severe bleeding on my return home. This book spells out in clear and concise language what parents need to know and how to prepare children for the surgery. Suggestions for how to talk to children in developmentally appropriate language will be especially helpful to parents. I enthusiastically recommend this book to parents of children facing this medical procedure and commend the Zelingers for writing such an immensely practical and useful book.

David A. Crenshaw, Ph.D., ABPP, Board Certified Clinical Psychologist,
Author, Clinical Director of the Children's Home of Poughkeepsie

Contents

Table of Figures

Dedicated to the Zelinger boys:

Jordan, Elliot, David, and Perry

Our four best reasons for learning how to ease a child through the difficult times in life.

Foreword

I have had the pleasure of knowing Dr. Laurie Zelinger through the care of her son. As a caring person involved with children, she brought her clinical insights into the office, especially when discussing her son.

Dr. Zelinger became interested in this project while preparing for her own son's surgery. She has had first-hand experience and decided to write to help prepare others for this significant life event. I believe she has addressed parental concerns and the way parents might best interact with their children to prepare them for these procedures.

She deserves a great deal of credit for the way she dealt with the needs of her own family, and especially her ability to transform that experience so that others might benefit.

Mark. N. Goldstein, M.D., P.C.
Fellow, American Academy of Otolaryngology
Fellow, American Academy of Pediatrics
Fellow, American College of Surgeons

Note: this Foreword was originally written in 2008 for the 1ˢᵗ Edition, formerly titled *The "O, MY" in Tonsillectomy and Adenoidectomy*. Dr. Goldstein passed away in 2014.

Preface to the 3rd Edition

This manual is intended as a guide toward navigating the preparation and surgical process that you and your child are about to undergo. The pronouns and particulars reflect those that pertained to our own situation. Please change them as needed to reflect your circumstances. If you do not have the luxury of several weeks for preparation, read through this manual in its entirety and select those recommendations that are practical for your lifestyle and timeframe, condensing and accelerating the suggestions to fit your schedule. This book was initially revised two years after its first printing, in response to readers' requests for information about possible yet unlikely and unexpected complications following surgery. Parents also requested information as to how they could talk with their other children about the process. It is being revised once again to reflect recent advances and changes in the medical approach toward tonsillectomies and adenoidectomies.

Laurie Zelinger, PhD and Perry Zelinger, MD

Uh-Oh, Surgery? Making Your Decision

Not again? You can't believe it! Your child was on antibiotics just a few weeks ago and now he has another sore throat. He keeps getting sick. Your pediatrician's office is closed and you're back at the urgent care center where the staff remember you and even greet you by your first name when you walk in. When the doctor's office calls you the next morning with the strep test results, they suggest that it is time to see a specialist. Or if

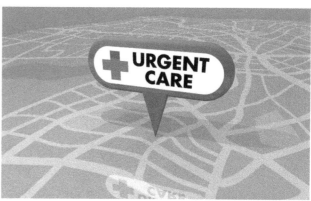

it isn't a sore throat that concerns you, perhaps you have a child who breathes through her mouth, snores at night and may gasp sometimes when she is sleeping. If either of these scenarios is familiar, you are probably heading for a consultation with an Otolaryngologist, better known as an Ear, Nose and Throat doctor, or ENT, for short.

As a responsible parent, you have made an appointment with a reputable ENT. During that visit, she reviewed the medical history, examined your child and then met with you in the consultation room to give you the news. Based on the frequency of your child's sore throats over the past year and/or other criteria established by the American Academy of Pediatrics and The American Academy of Otolaryngology-Head and Neck Surgery, the Ear Nose and Throat doctor is now recommending surgery to remove your child's tonsils and/or adenoids. While complete surgical removal (tonsillectomy) is the most common approach for remediation, partial removal (tonsillotomy) is

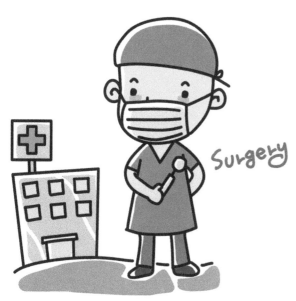

gaining popularity based on faster postoperative recovery time and reduced pain. Partial removal however, carries with it the small chance of tissue re-growth that sometimes requires a repeat procedure (Walton, Ebner, Stewart & April, 2012). Removal of the tonsils helps to address infections that are caused by substances entering the mouth, whereas adenoid removal addresses those germs which have entered through the nose and might cause nasal obstruction, ear or sinus infections and snoring.

Oh, so much to think about. So what do you do? Get the facts!

From a historical perspective, the number of tonsillectomies performed in the United States to combat infection has declined dramatically over time, while surgery for reasons of obstruction has increased. There were nearly one million tonsillectomies reported in 1965 for children under age 15, yet by 2010 that total reached only 289,000; one third higher in girls than boys. Likewise, adenoidectomies for that age group declined by nearly half during the four-year period from 2006 to 2010, dropping from 132,000 to 69,000 (Paradise & Wald, 2018) with a rate 1.5 times higher in boys. Although tonsillectomies and adenoidectomies can be performed separately, they are often performed together in a procedure referred to as *adenotonsillectomy* (AT), occurring at an annual rate of 500,000 in the United States at the current time (Garetz, 2018). Most tonsillectomies for children over age three years are performed in an outpatient setting, and children often go home just a few hours after the procedure. Adenotonsillectomies account for the second most common outpatient surgical procedure performed on children in the United States, following after myringotomy, which is ear tube placement (Hall, Schwartzman, Zhang, & Liu, 2018).

Sleep Disordered Breathing

The two most common reasons by far for childhood adenotonsillectomies are sleep-disordered breathing (SDB) and recurrent infections, although enlarged tonsils can also lead to inability to swallow properly as well as voice and speech deviations such as tongue thrusts and inter-dental lisps. If you are reading this book, chances are that your child is experiencing one of these issues, prompting your appointment with an Ear, Nose and Throat specialist to evaluate her condition.

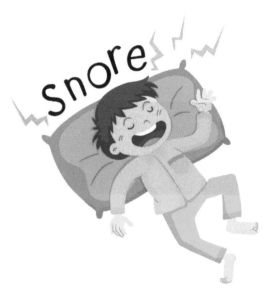

Sleep Disordered Breathing, peaking in children between the ages of two and eight, is the general term that includes problems such as simple snoring and Obstructive Sleep Apnea (OSA). This condition is due to restricted airflow during the night, which can result in gasping, restlessness or arousal from sleep and is associated with lower concentrations of oxygen and higher levels of carbon dioxide in the blood (Garetz, 2018). To formally diagnose OSA, an overnight sleep study known as polysomnography is required, but this is often unnecessary unless children present with particular risk factors for postoperative respiratory complications. Even though Sleep Disordered Breathing is technically the correct term, you may hear the term Obstructive Sleep Apnea used interchangeably; they are the same.

It is important to understand that adenotonsillectomy is done not only to address snoring; obstructive sleep apnea is also associated with behavioral problems resembling Attention Deficit Hyperactivity Disorder (ADHD), poor academic school performance, bedwetting, and growth failure. All of these may improve after tonsillectomy. If left untreated, OSA can also lead to cardiac issues, high blood pressure, continued cognitive and behavioral problems, and may significantly affect quality of life (Baugh, Archer, Mitchell, et al., 2011). Removal of enlarged adenoids and tonsils is considered the first-line treatment for sleep disordered breathing in children over the age of two. (Paradise & Wald, 2018 and Garetz, 2018).

Recurrent Infections

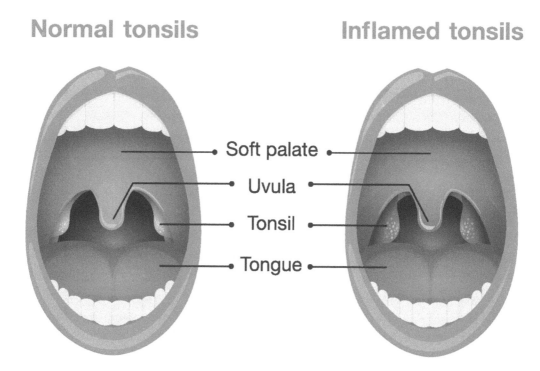

Fig. 1: Normal vs. Inflamed Tonsils

The second indication for surgery, mentioned earlier, is to address recurrent infections. Adeno-tonsillectomy is not recommended routinely for every child who experiences sore throats. Rather, frequency and severity of those episodes are taken into account. A child may be a candidate for surgery if he has had either of these:

- More than 7 infections in the past year, 5 each year for past 2 years, or 3 per year for past 3 years.
- Clinical features such as oral temperature over 101 Fahrenheit (or 38.3 Celsius), and a return of infections despite more conservative prior treatment with antibiotics for one month and nasal steroids for six weeks (Paradise & Wald, 2018).

While these guidelines are widely recognized, some children may not fully meet these criteria and may be treated with watchful waiting instead. (Baugh, et al., 2011; Garetz, 2018).

Alternative options for OSA include Continuous Positive Airway Pressure (CPAP) for pediatric sleep apnea, weight loss, and/or rapid maxillary expansion, which is an orthodontic procedure using a palate expander to widen the palate and nasal passages in order to increase airway availability and reduce obstruction.

In addition to the two primary indicators of sleep disordered breathing and infection, there are other lesser common reasons to get adenotonsillectomy that include voice abnormalities, tonsil area abscess, trouble swallowing, dental issues, unremitting bad breath, and some other rare disorders. Your ENT has taken all of this information into account and has probably made a recommendation. Now that the examination visit is over, you may have a decision to make. Oh my! Where do you go from here?

After the Consult

As you leave the Otolaryngologist's office, you are flooded with emotions and information. Maybe your child even overheard some of the conversation at the doctor's office. What do you do first? You have an option to schedule surgery on the spot, or to go home and sort things out. Our suggestion is to defer any decision until you and your partner, or other trusted person, can speak comfortably and privately. Do not discuss this topic on the car ride home. Children do not need to hear both sides of the situation, or any concerns you may have. The message they must get is that you (both) wholeheartedly endorse the decision you have reached, and that there is no room for doubt or change of mind.

Never assume that your child is too young to understand what you might discuss. Even if the words are not fully understood, your tone of voice and gestures will convey your feelings. Wait until you are alone to discuss your options. If your child asks what will be happening, reassure him that nothing is happening yet. The doctor visit is over, and now you are going home (or wherever). You might say that Mommy and Daddy and the Ear/Nose/Throat (ENT) doctor are all working together to figure out the best way to help his throat and ears to feel better. This explanation should be enough to quell any immediate concerns. Then, use the next few days to think about the recommendations, and speak with your pediatrician. You may even want to get a second opinion.

Preparation begins for you and your child once you have actually scheduled surgery. Read everything you are given about the procedure, until you feel that most of your own questions have been answered. Then, and only then, can you begin to prepare your child.

Phase 1: Introducing the Topic to Your Child

1 to 2 Months before Surgery

You may want to ask your ENT doctor to recommend a child's book for you to read to your youngster, or you may find a suitable YouTube video. The reference list at the back of this book suggests some sources to consider.

At some reasonable time before the surgery (several weeks if you have the luxury of time), leave the book within your child's reach to casually investigate. After you have noticed some interest, begin to read it to your youngster for the first time. You probably will not have a chance to get through the entire story. Every few days, begin to read it over again from the beginning, trying to add a paragraph or page at each new reading. The aim is to familiarize your child at his own pace. Stop reading if your child becomes upset. Put it down for a few days and try again at some other point. Whatever amount you accomplish at this point is fine, since your goal is just to set the stage for future discussion.

Several weeks before surgery, indicate to your child that one day, but not yet, he will have his tonsils out too, just like the child in the book. Then he will feel better (i.e., not have to be absent from school and be able to sleep better at night). Be specific about the improvement of his particular recurring symptoms.

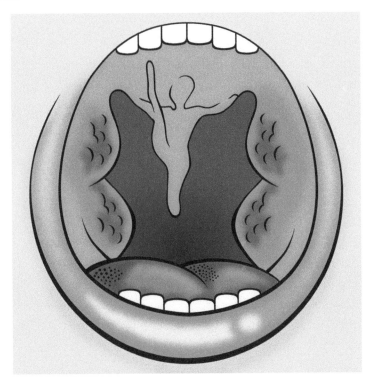

Fig. 2: Uvula as an acrobat– illustration for children

A Child-Friendly Explanation

Your child may ask you what tonsils and adenoids are. You can share the fanciful uvula picture on the previous page and say something similar to the explanation in the box below:

> Lots of parts of our bodies have special jobs. Just like our legs are for walking, our nose is for smelling and our tongue is for tasting, our tonsils have a job too. We have two of them way back in our mouth, by our throat. If we open our mouth wide, and look in with a flashlight, it sort of looks like a stage with the lights off before a show. There is a thing hanging down in the middle. It's called a uvula, and it's like an acrobat who is hanging from the ceiling on the stage. If we look to the sides, we'll see a pink bump on each side that looks like the curtain. Those bumps are the tonsils. Their job is to help our body fight sickness and infection by catching germs that come into our body. When the tonsils get full of germs and stop working well, they are not doing their job and we end up getting sick. Lots of times, the doctor will say that if we get rid of sick tonsils, the rest of our body will feel better.
>
> Another part of our body that has a job like the tonsils is called the adenoids. They're behind the stage, so they're too far back to see when we look in our mouth. When the adenoids get sick, they get bigger and take up a lot of room in our mouth. If we have big tonsils and big adenoids, they take up a lot of space and then it's sometimes hard to breathe. When that happens, we breathe loudly in the daytime, and we snore at night.
>
> But if we take out these parts with all the germs in them, we will breathe more easily and feel better. Those parts of our body are extra and we don't need them. There are special doctors who know just the right way to take out tonsils, since a gazillion kids need to get rid of theirs. Mommy and Daddy called a lot of doctors and found just the right one we liked the best. His name is Dr. (*insert your surgeon's name here*), and he will help your mouth and throat get better."

Once you have selected the date and place for surgery, determine where it falls within a timeframe your child can understand, and create a calendar you can refer to. Then use that personal frame of reference in all your future mentions (e.g., "Your tonsils aren't coming out yet. We will go back to Dr. ENT (after winter vacation, after your birthday, when camp starts, etc.") By linking the date of surgery to a personal reference point or major event, your child will be able to gain a more concrete understanding of its occurrence while allaying his fears of an immediate procedure. It will also allow for ample opportunities to bring it up whenever you talk about the holiday, birthday, etc. preceding it. At this point, you should not give a drawn-out explanation, but merely a mention of it when the opportunity presents itself.

Within a few weeks, you should be able to ask your child what will happen after Grandma comes to visit (or whatever you have selected as your personal reference point), and his response should become an automatic reply about tonsils, even though he will not yet fully understand the procedure. That's okay at this stage. Use the words, "tonsils" and "adenoids" as often as you can because the more you do, the more you are helping your child to become desensitized to what is likely to be a frightening situation. The more chances he has to talk or to think about it, the more it will inevitably help him to better deal with the procedure. Playing out the procedure using dolls or puppets and a toy medical kit will give your child the opportunity to express her feelings as well as to recognize what questions or worries she may have. The classic Milton Bradley board game

"Operation" (now sold by Hasbro) also introduces the theme of removing and fixing ailing body parts.

You may want to make a simple calendar indicating the personal reference point and the date of surgery, so that you can cross off the days as they draw near. This will also help your child to feel more in control, since children are in a vulnerable situation where only the grown-ups get to call (and give!) the shots.

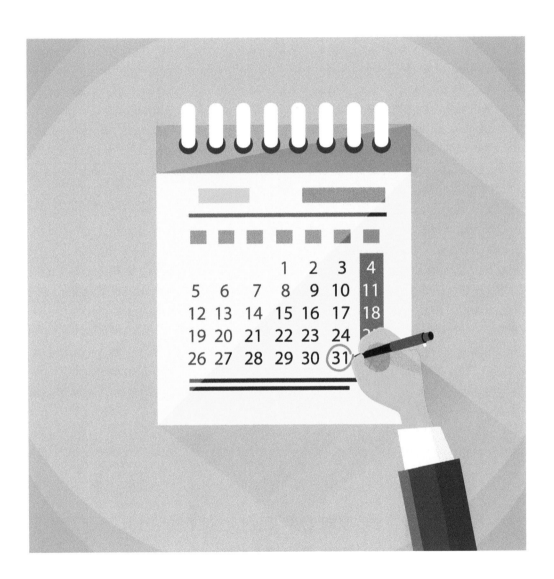

Fig. 3: Using your calendar to organize the surgery schedule

Phase 2: Tackling the Subject

What to Tell Your Child 3 to 4 Weeks before Surgery

About 3 weeks before surgery, your descriptions and references to the procedure will increase. By now, you will have made several attempts to read your selected book. If you have been unsuccessful until now, set aside time free of distraction for both of you, and read it aloud, even if your child becomes fearful. At this point, read a little more, even through the tears, but keep reassuring him that surgery will not take place until after the personal reference time you have selected. Experts believe that anxiety diminishes as you are able to get mental or physical exposure to the feared event. And research shows that those children whose anxiety was highest before surgery experienced more pain during recovery (Messner, 2018). Furthering the discussion now is necessary, and should not be avoided at the child's first sign of discomfort.

Read and talk slowly, and be careful to stay calm when your child protests. Let your child know that you understand what he is feeling. Say something like, "This seems very scary for you." Reassure your child that you will help him to become less afraid (i.e., "Mommy will be there with you the whole time, and will hold you. We'll be together. Maybe we'll even bring your teddy bear.")

Don't try to talk your child out of what she is feeling. She is afraid, and telling her not to be will only make her think that you don't understand. Trying to choose the right words to say is not as important as conveying the gentle tone and message that you understand and are trying to do everything you can to help. Let your child know that she can talk about her worries any time she thinks of them. You also want to give the message to all of your children that sick tonsils are not caused by anyone's behavior or anything a child thinks about or wishes. Children can't make someone need a tonsillectomy.

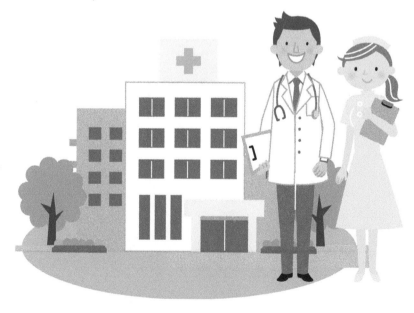

What to Tell Your Child 2 to 3 Weeks before Surgery

Most people wilt when they hear the words "operation" or "hospital." They have an image in their mind, formed by personal experience, which is frequently exaggerated by "horror" stories or graphic portrayals seen on television. It is your mission to avoid creating these associations for your child. Instead of using the word "operation," describe simply that Dr. ENT will "take out" his tonsils because they have been hurting and you want him to feel better. Rather than using the word "hospital," describe it as Dr. ENT's "other" office at the Day-Op, Outpatient or Medical Center. Referring to Dr. ENT by name reduces the mystery and the tendency for your child to invent information. Your child has already had contact with her and has established a frame of reference. An office is a place where children have frequently seen doctors and nurses, and is far less intimidating in one's imagination than a hospital would be.

You may choose to call the operating room a "special room" where the doctor has all the things he needs to fix tonsils, and the term "resting room," because after surgery (in recovery), that is indeed what your child will do. However, if your child is already familiar with other terminology, do not deny the correct terms. The idea is to help your child conceptualize the experience in advance by describing the sequence of events in terms she can understand.

To put this all together as your first explanation to your child, find a time during which you will not be disturbed and when your child is most likely to be responsive to you; not while he's watching TV or waiting with bated breath for a playmate to come over. Earlier in the day would be best, as it allows you time to think about the experience and ask questions as they arise. Introduce the topic with reference to the book (which you have now completed together at least once), or by asking what will be happening after (your personal reference point). When your child responds that his tonsils /adenoids will come out, that is your opportunity to take the conversation further.

Ask what he remembers. Then tell him what the day will probably be like. He may stop you several times to talk about something else, or may ask for vivid details about any one procedure. If you don't know the answer to a question, be honest and say so. Tell your child that he asked a great question and you will try to find out the answer. Then make it your business to do so. Even if your child does not seem particularly attentive, try to describe, even superficially, what he can expect on the day of surgery. He is probably absorbing some of the information and taking in what he is able to handle at the time. This might be a good opportunity to play with dolls and a medical kit, puppets or the Milton-Bradley game "Operation" (*without* the batteries) to acquaint your youngster with the experience.

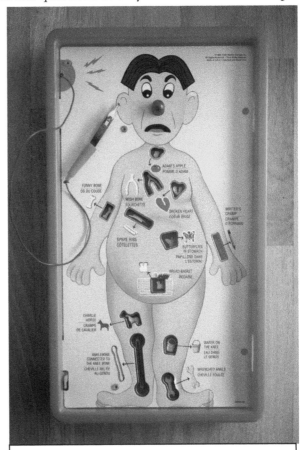

Fig. 4: "Operation" teaches important concepts

By now, you will also have some idea as to who will be accompanying your child to the medical center. Ideally, two adults (with whom he is most comfortable) should go so that one can attend to the child while the other completes the necessary paperwork. Keep in mind that usually only ONE parent will be allowed into the operating suite. Decide ahead of time whom that will be, if indeed you feel that one of you can be there without getting upset. Having two adults at the medical center also allows one person to sit at the child's bedside during recovery, while the other person takes a break. If you are a single parent, perhaps you can bring an aunt, uncle or grandparent to stay for even just part of the time. If possible arrange for somebody else to be responsible for transportation back home. That way you would have the opportunity to sit in the back seat next to your child while someone else drives. Then tell some version of the following scenario and vary it as you see fit for your youngster, personalizing it for your own situation

Explaining it all to your 3 to 7-year-old child:

> On the day when your tonsils come out, you will wake up and watch TV like always (or do what you typically do in the morning). Then you will get dressed and can play a little, but we won't have breakfast on that day. After we play, we're going to go in Daddy's car and drive to Dr. ENT's other office at the Day-Op Center. Remember, we saw that place already? (Refer to Phase 3 in this manual). When we get there, you and Daddy can play in the playroom while Mommy fills out papers and talks to the woman in the office.
>
> When they call our name, we'll go into a little room and a doctor or nurse will look in your ears and nose and mouth and listen to your heart with a stethoscope (see Fig. 5).

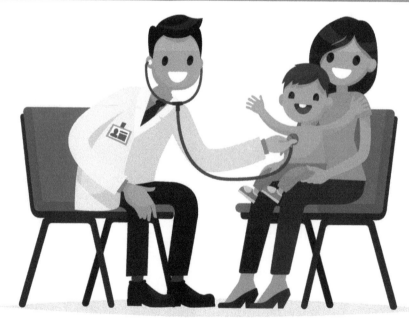

Fig. 5: Doctor examining with Stethoscope

Remember what that is? Dr. (*your pediatrician's name*) wears that around his neck and puts it on your back and chest when he listens to you breathe. The nurse at the Day-Op Center will take your temperature and blood pressure with that squeezy thing they put around your arm and will probably do some other things that nurses do.

Then we'll go into another office and they will give us different clothes. You can go into a bathroom or dressing room to change. You'll take off your shoes and socks and pants and shirt and underwear. (Some children get very upset at removing their underwear. If you expect that to be the case, speak to the nurse.) They will give you a costume like a soft pillow case (it's called a gown) that we will tie closed, and maybe even special socks that'll keep you warm and keep you from slipping when you walk. The nurse will also give you a plastic bracelet to wear that will have your name on it and some numbers. And Mommy will have to put on a special costume also. Then we'll wait again. We might even see other people in the same kind of gown who are waiting, too. And we'll see doctors and nurses who will be wearing special clothes and even a puffy kind of hat so their hair won't get in the way when they work. Dr. ENT will come out and say hello to us.

A little while after that, you might get on a riding toy and drive it right into the "special room" while mommy walks with you, or we can carry you. There will be a lot of people in there who are Dr. ENT's helpers, and they will all be wearing the same kind of clothes and maybe a matching cover over their mouth so they can't give us germs if they cough or sneeze. But we'll be able to see their eyes, and when they crinkle, we'll know they are smiling underneath.

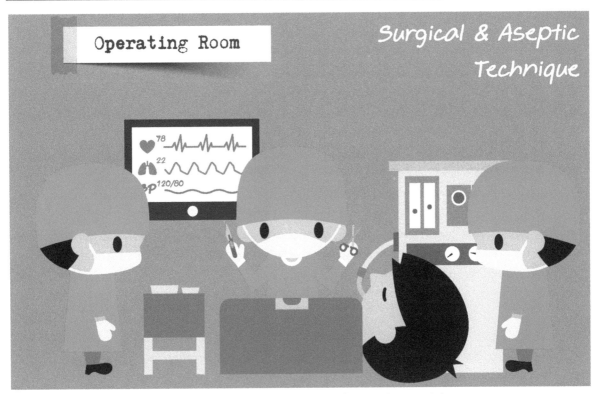

Fig. 6: Silver machines and bright lights in the special room

There will be a lot of silver machines and bright lights in the 'special room,' (see Fig. 6) everyone will be busy and it will feel cold, since the air conditioner will be on. You'll climb onto a skinny silver table and will lie on your back, or you might sit on Mommy's lap. Mommy will sit on a chair right next to the table and will hold your hand. Then Mommy will give you an astronaut's mask to breathe from that the nurse will hold over your nose and mouth. Sometimes you get to decide what kind of smell you would like the air in the mask to have. After a little while it will make you feel sleepy, like you are floating. Mommy will stay there until you fall asleep and you will stay asleep until it's all over. You won't feel anything.

When you wake up (see Fig. 6), you will be in a different bed and you'll see a nurse first, before you see Mommy or Daddy. You'll feel different and your nose and mouth will feel scratchy and will hurt. You'll probably be shivering for a little while. Your stomach might not feel so good either. You might feel like throwing up, but you will feel better later. Then Mommy and Daddy will come to see you and wait with you while you take a nap. Other children may be taking a nap also in the same room. When you wake up, your arm may be resting on a board and it may have tape on it. The tape is holding a tube in place that's called "IV" and looks like a long skinny tube from a fish tank. At the other end of the tube is a see-through bag that will be hanging on a silver pole right next to your bed. That bag has special medicine and vitamins in it to make you feel better faster.

A different nurse will come to visit you and examine you. She will ask you what you like to drink or what kind of ices you like to eat. You'll feel a little cranky, but if you eat and drink stuff, and make urine ("pee-pee," "sissy"), they will let us know when you can go home. When you're ready, Mommy will help you get your own clothes on and you'll be wheeled to the door in a chair with big wheels on it. Then we'll go back home in Daddy's car. If you're not ready to go home yet, the doctors might say that they want you sleep over so they can check you the next day to make sure everything is just right.

When you get home, you will sleep a lot and you may get mixed up whether it's daytime or nighttime. You will have to stay in bed for a while and can only play quiet games. People might send you cards or presents and everyone will ask how you feel. Your voice will be very low for a few days and will probably sound different. Sometimes you will feel good and sometimes you will feel bad. But medicine will help you feel better. You will stay home from school for a lot of days and your voice will probably sound funny for a while. Then, after seven days, you will visit Dr. ENT and he'll look in your mouth. It will not hurt. He will tell you when you can go out and play and when you can eat pizza again and when you can go back to school. By then you will have a lot of energy and will feel like doing everything you used to do. You will be all better and will not get sick so much anymore. You will feel happier and will probably grow a lot and get bigger very fast.

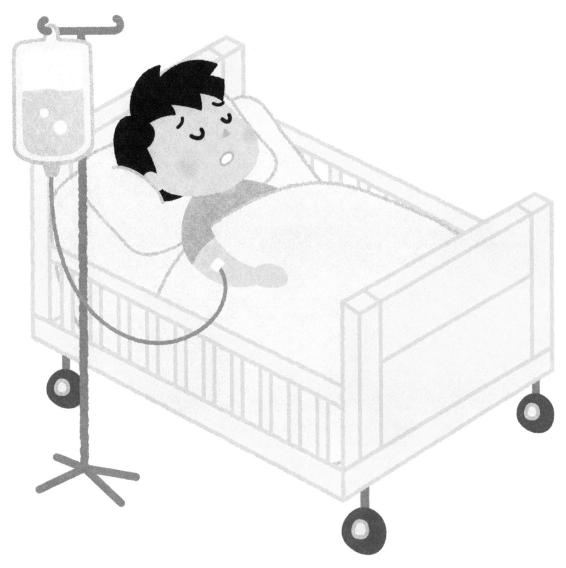

Fig. 7: Resting in the recovery room

Phase 3: Getting Closer, Getting Ready

1 to 2 Weeks to Go

You and your child should be having frequent talks about the surgery by now. Involve him in preparing for those long days at home to follow the surgery. Now that you have some time, take him shopping with you. Let your child choose his favorite flavor of Jell-o, yogurt, ice cream, sorbet, pudding, nectar or variety of pasta and creamed cereal. Allow him to select the potatoes that will be cooked for mashed potatoes. Even though he may be long past baby food, many children enjoy permission to eat jarred baby food again. Although there are few dietary restrictions following surgery, it is wise to avoid the tart fruit varieties and all textured foods for the first few days. You will also need plenty of drinks. Sodas are acceptable if you stir them first to release the bubbles. Be lenient with nutrition rules during the post-operative week. Your goal is to keep your child swallowing anything he can manage and drinking is more important than eating. Buy plastic straws and let him help you cut 3 inches off the bottom (shorter straws require less effort for drinking). Pick up interesting cups with different colors, themes, covers, sizes, etc., as well as plain lollipops without filling. Buy a strip thermometer that can be placed on his forehead, since some children have pain in their ears following this procedure and may not tolerate anything placed in their ear. Your child will probably have difficulty using an oral thermometer now, and the invasive nature of a rectal thermometer may cause added anxiety following surgery. You will probably be instructed not to give your child any pain relievers containing ibuprofen for two weeks prior to his surgery.

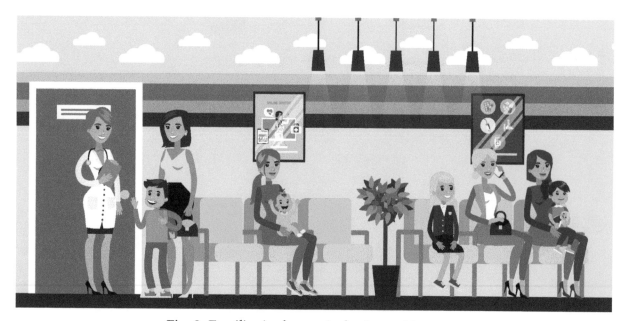

Fig. 8: Families in the surgical suite waiting room

Arrange to visit the medical center where the surgery will take place, either as part of a tour or on your own. Take your child on a leisurely stroll through the waiting room, playroom and bathroom. Eat a snack there. Make a phone call, or drink from the water fountain. Watch people coming and going. Stay long enough (15-30 minutes) to help your child form a memory of it and to see enough to talk about. Draw a picture or take a photo of it while you are there, or play "I spy something with my little eye" (to do that, you each take turns locating something in the room and the other person must guess what you are thinking of). Do not leave until you see that your child is habituating and is less anxious than when you arrived. Psychologists refer to this in-vivo experience as Exposure with Response Prevention (Rowa, Antony & Swinson, 2007). You may even use this opportunity to explore the facility if you go there for your lab work one week before surgery.

If you have a good relationship with your dentist, you may want to visit his office to try on the nitrous oxide mask in advance, (without the gas) reassuring your youngster that the dentist is not looking in her mouth. Let your child feel it, take it on and off, get acquainted with the idea of something over her nose like astronauts use. The actual mask used during surgery will cover her mouth also, however this visit to the dentist is only meant to introduce your child to what she will experience so there are fewer surprises. You may need to reassure other children in the family that this procedure is not happening to them and to give them an explanation of the procedure. Depending upon the ages of your other children, you may want to tell them something along these lines:

> You know how your sister is always getting sore throats? That's because her tonsils keep getting sick. Dr. (pediatrician's name) told us that if we can get rid of her sick tonsils, she will feel a lot better, so we want to do that. We'll go to a special doctor who will take them out. On that day, Mommy and I will leave early and Grandma will be watching you. When we come home, your sister will be very tired and won't feel so well. Mommy and I will need to give her a lot of attention for a few days, until she starts to feel better. But we can still take care of you too, because we love all of you the same amount, and grandma will help if we get very busy. Since your sister may need to sleep a lot, we'll have to be quiet sometimes. If that's hard for you, we can set up some play dates at your friend's house. Even though your sister is having her tonsils out, that doesn't mean that you will. All kids are different.

You may have to cancel some of your responsibilities and arrange to take time off from work for those important few days after surgery when your child may be feeling miserable. This will remind your child how important she is to you.

3 to 7 Days to Go

One week before surgery, your child will need to have necessary and specific lab (blood) work performed. This can be done at an independent laboratory or at the medical center where surgery will be performed. If you expect that the blood test may be particularly upsetting, consider having it done in an independent setting so as not to establish the surgical site as a place to be feared. Ask your pediatrician if he will be requiring any routine blood work within the near future that could be drawn at the same time, since schools and camps sometimes require lab work for their programs. This might avoid putting your child through additional blood testing in the pediatrician's office at his next well-visit checkup.

Go to the library and borrow books to read during the recuperation week. Gather all toys that can be used in bed and store them nearby in one place. Quiet games like a deck of cards, Lite-Brite™, Etch A Sketch™ or Magna Doodle™, puzzles, Pick Up Sticks, arts and crafts, Play-Doh™, shape sorters, beads, Woodkins Dress-Up Kids™, Mr. Potato Head™, Legos™, Scratch Art, board games and lanyard are among the many quiet activities that can occupy your child. Remove the "too active" toys from his view to avoid frustration. You might even move the TV into his room temporarily, buy little gifts or borrow new videos that can be given when something extra is needed to boost his spirits or break the monotony. Make an audio recording of a bedtime story at your next regular reading. Your child will revel in hearing himself interposed during the story, and you can play it during those post-operative days of bed rest. Your child might appreciate having a bell to ring when he needs you. Set up a daybed and night bed in different rooms if possible, so your child has a change of scenery and cool sheets when he's ready for nighttime sleep. Move a cot into your room for your child, or one into the child's room for you. Use a baby monitor or intercom so he won't have to call you when he needs something. Schedule a clearance check-up with the pediatrician for the day before surgery.

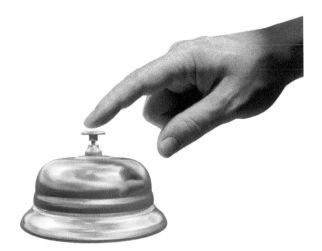

Fig. 9: Set up a bell or baby monitor

Counting Down the Days: 3-2-1

Stay calm. Keep your child indoors, and away from other children for a few days before surgery to avoid getting sick (i.e., no birthday parties, school or other crowded areas).

Bring your child to the pediatrician for clearance in order to proceed with surgery, and ask the doctor to give you a letter to present to the surgeon. If your child is sick, surgery will probably be postponed. A window of three weeks is usually considered safe after an episode of acute infection and before surgery in order to guard against the risk of excessive bleeding during the procedure (Paradise & Wald, 2018). In the event that surgery gets postponed, tell your child that being sick means he has germs (i.e., in his throat). Since germs aren't allowed in the "special" room, it is necessary to wait to get his tonsils out until he is better.

Fill all prescriptions for post-surgical medications one day in advance, if possible. Have several medicine dispensers available. Squirting types tend to reduce the need for the child to strain his neck by tilting back to drink from a cup or from a flow-type dispenser. Create a chart to keep track of when you give your child his medications. You may want to ask your child's teacher to send some work home that you can do together toward the end of the week.

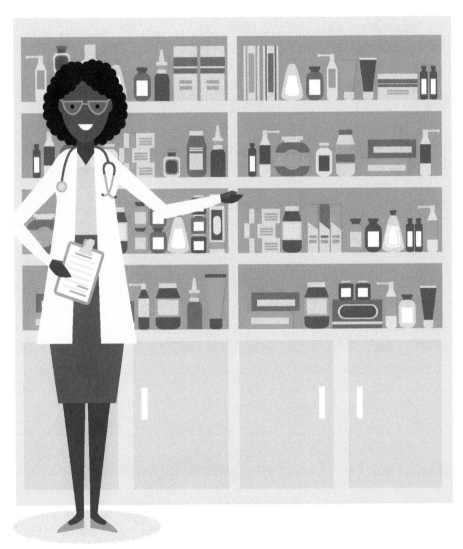

Fig. 10: Fill all prescriptions for post-surgical medications in advance if possible

Phase 4: The Day of Surgery- It's Here!

On the Morning of Surgery

You should wake up early enough to eat breakfast, shower and get dressed before waking your child. Take care of the needs of other family members before waking the patient. Change the morning routine slightly so that your child will not come to expect breakfast at the usual time, since he will not be permitted to eat or drink anything from midnight the night before. Not even chewing gum.

Pack the following items: the medical clearance letter from your pediatrician and insurance cards, an extra front-opening shirt so that your child will not have to strain his neck to get on a pullover; a favorite comforting device (e.g. teddy bear, blanket); a DVD, video, laptop or iPad loaded with your child's favorite movies, because the guest Wi-Fi might be inaccessible or limited; a distraction for yourself (book, crossword puzzle) enough snacks for you for a six-hour stay, contact information for family members or babysitters, and a cell phone charger. In the unlikely event that your child is not permitted to go home that day, an overnight bag with clothes and supplies for both of you should be prepared and left in the car, "just in case." Leave all get-well gifts at home. Your child will be too groggy to enjoy them. Put a blanket, pillow, baby wipes and stomach-sickness bag in the car for the ride home.

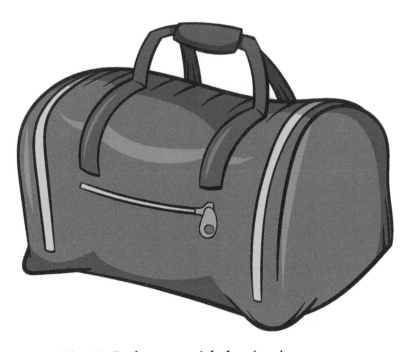

Fig. 11: Pack an overnight bag just in case

During Surgery

If you are able, accompany your child into the operating room. He may ride a motorized vehicle there or perhaps you might carry him in and help him climb onto the table. Be as relaxed and reassuring as possible to your child. He may be frightened and need to focus on you, especially since the rest of the team will be wearing masks and only your voice and face will be recognizable. You might even be allowed to hold him in your lap. Sometimes you are given the option to hold the anesthesia mask over his nose and mouth. As you do so, tell his favorite story in a quiet, calm and slow voice. Continue to make your voice softer as the anesthesia begins to take effect. Be prepared for an agitation phase, when your child may thrash a little under the mask and the pupils of his eyes will become dilated. It may be upsetting to you, but it indicates deepening sedation. Stroke his hair and remind him of your presence. Then leave the operating room when you are asked to do so. Expect to wait almost an hour for an AT procedure. You will be reunited in the recovery room. Often, only one parent at a time is permitted into the recovery room immediately afterward.

Immediately After Surgery in the Recovery Room

Your child will be disoriented. While his eyes may be open, he may not seem to focus or recognize you. Your child may be in a dream-like state for up to an hour, even though he is awake. It can be very upsetting to a parent to see a child in an incoherent state and not able to relate to you. This is an aftereffect of general anesthesia and will wear off with the passing of time. He may also have dried blood around his mouth, since tonsils are removed through the mouth, not through an incision in the skin. If he is able to talk, he may repeat the same questions over and over and may speak at a different rate than usual. He may shiver, cry, sleep or throw up and will probably feel cold.

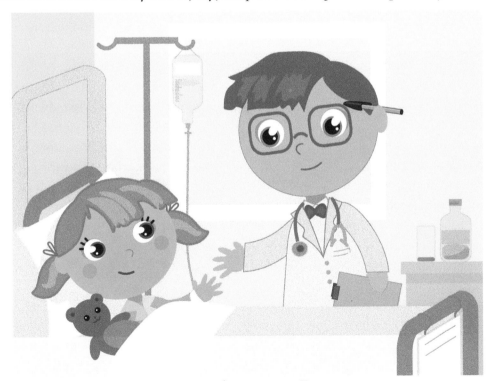

Fig. 12: In the Recovery Room

He may want you nearby, or to go away, or both. Be patient. His behavior will not be predictable, and for a while he may seem like a different child. The constriction of lying on his side to prevent inhaling residual blood and the limited mobility from the intravenous tubes will also be frustrating, and your child may even succeed in dislodging some of the paraphernalia. There is little you can do during this difficult period but to wait with your child and to remain as calm as possible. Let him see you. Tell him where he is and that his tonsils are already out. Keep your sentences short and simple, and don't ask questions that require answers. Force fluids, since drinking is essential. You should expect to be in the recovery area for about four hours, although 2-10 hours is common, and you will most likely be sharing space with other families in the same position. Your child's vital signs will be monitored at regular intervals. Fluid intake and output standards (in a bedpan) must be met before you can all go home. In the unlikely event of a known or unforeseen complication, or if your child is under three years of age, they may be required to stay longer for observation and/or and treatment. Some surgeons estimate that 10 percent of their patients stay overnight. If that should occur, you may want to give your child an explanation and these words might help:

> Your tonsils are finally out and you're on your way to getting better. Dr. ENT sometimes likes to watch children sleep after their tonsils come out to make sure they're ready to go home. We are going to have a sleep over here together tonight, and some nurses will take care of us. Tomorrow, Dr. ENT will look in your mouth again and will tell us when we can go home."

At Home after Surgery

It is a tremendous relief to be home, but you may worry about recuperation. Ear, neck and throat pain, especially upon swallowing, may persist for 7-14 days, which might reduce your child's willingness to drink. It is critical to maintain his fluid intake and limit vomiting in order to prevent dehydration, which could otherwise lead to a trip to the Emergency Department. The anesthesiologist has likely administered medication during anesthesia to help reduce nausea in the Recovery Room, but there are also medications the doctor can prescribe to help alleviate nausea at home. Pain, which is usually reported to be worse in the morning than the evening, is often safely controlled with acetaminophen or ibuprofen on an as-needed basis; whereas aspirin and opioids are usually contraindicated because of the increased bleeding risk they might pose (Messner, 2018).

Keep your physician's phone number handy in the event that you have any concerns. Your phone call will not be an imposition. Write down all of your questions so that you don't forget to ask any. Keep a pen handy to write the answers. Tape your post-operative instruction sheet to a wall near your child's bed, near the phone or on the refrigerator. Additionally, keep a chart of the times you administer each medication.

Expect everybody's sleep patterns to be altered. With frequent napping, day and night times may get confused. Some children have nightmares as a result of the anesthesia or the trauma of the actual event. This will improve as recuperation progresses. Nausea may be another effect of general anesthesia, plaguing your child for the next few days unless your physician has prescribed an anti-emetic. Keep a waste basket nearby to avoid the need to run to the bathroom, and cold compresses applied to the back of the neck sometimes helps relieve nausea. Your child may experience

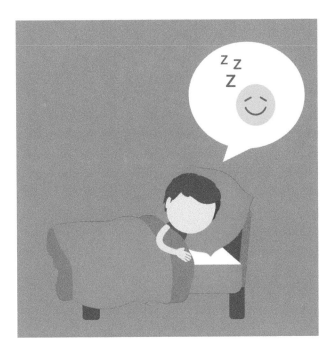

swallowing difficulties. It will be painful, and sometimes when they drink, liquid may move up into the nose as the body readjusts to the changes and increased space in the throat. When your child awakens from sleep, there may be some dried blood on her lips. Use a RED washcloth to wipe away (and camouflage) any signs of minor bleeding. Additional pillows should be used to keep her head elevated, and colorful, print pillowcases will detract from stains caused by post-operative oozing. Refrigerate medication to ease in its swallowing. Cold liquids will help to reduce swelling and numb the area. In addition, gargling with ¼ teaspoon of salt in 8 ounces of warm water is encouraged, and saline nasal sprays are often recommended for nasal stuffiness or secretions. Bad breath is common and expected, and may last up to two weeks.

Allow your child special privileges, since nothing is ordinary about her recent experience. Restrict traffic in the house to avoid excitement and the tendency to be active too quickly, as well as to avoid contact with others who may be carrying germs. Inform his teacher of the surgery so that classmates can make a get-well card. Use your toy medical kit and dolls or puppets to allow your child to act out the recent experience. Play with your child, making sure to do her favorite activities. Take a photo for future reference.

The first three days after surgery are the most difficult, and increased pain is sometimes reported on the fifth day, with scabs forming between five and ten days after surgery. However, significant improvement will follow over the next few weeks. It is easy to be fooled into thinking that your child is almost better when he shows interest in resuming activities and begins to feel less pain, but do NOT take him out prematurely! Vigorous activity can result in increased bleeding from dislodged scabs and may even lengthen the recuperation process. Follow your doctor's advice even if you think that your child is recovering more quickly than expected. Your child will probably return to school in about one week, and will probably be able to return to physical education class and sports within two. Since recuperation is a very individual process, comparisons among children should be avoided and existing concerns should be raised only with your doctor.

Over the next few months, you may notice several changes in your child. You may see rapid growth in height and weight, a renewed appetite and interest in food, and a change in the quality of his voice and speech. Resistance to ear, nose and throat infections will improve. Many parents even report improvement in their child's general disposition. While the experience will have undoubtedly been a difficult one for the whole family, children are resilient and bounce back quickly. Their successful journey through pre- and post-surgery will largely be the result of your preparation and effort. They will have you to thank for helping them to cope with what otherwise might have been a terrifying and overwhelming experience. Your child has succeeded in dealing with a difficult situation, learning that he has a foundation to deal with other challenges that come his way.

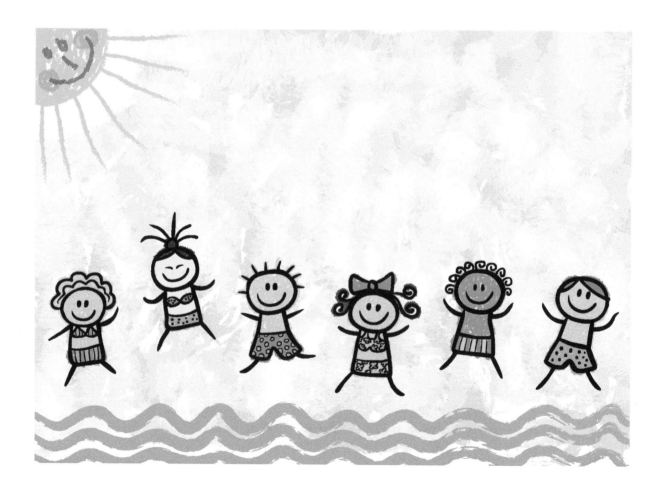

The Ultimate Preparation List

- Medical insurance information and pre-approval authorization letter
- Copy of the pediatrician's medical clearance (for surgery) letter
- Phone numbers for surgeon, pediatrician and pharmacy
- A children's book about tonsillectomies
- Several medicine dispensers
- Thermometer (ear or forehead strip)
- Prescription medications
- Pain relievers/Acetaminophen and ibuprofen
- Salt for gargling
- Saline nasal sprays
- Straws
- Drinks (plenty!) Give apple juice, Gatorade™ or Powerade™, grape juice or instant breakfast drinks, smoothies. *Avoid acidic juices such as orange or pineapple or fizzy drinks.*
- Baby food, scrambled eggs, pastina, farina, flavored ices, Jell-O™, yogurt, pudding, apple sauce, favorite soft foods. *Avoid sour, salty, hot, sharp or spicy foods.*
- Bell for child to ring if he needs you
- Baby monitor or intercom
- Red washcloths
- Extra pillows for elevation with printed pillow cases
- Quiet games/books for recuperation period
- Videos, iPad, tablet or other entertainment device
- USB chargers and cords for all devices carried
- Toy medical kit and dolls to represent patient and doctor
- "Operation" game by Milton Bradley (batteries not required)
- Set up a day and night bed in different locations
- Calendar
- Create a medication chart
- Make clearance appointment with pediatrician before surgery
- Make appointment with dentist to see nitrous oxide mask
- Front opening shirt to wear home after procedure
- Coins or pre-paid phone card for public telephones at surgical center
- Pillow and car sickness bag for ride home from surgery
- Overnight bag with clothing and essentials for you and your child, just in case he needs to spend the night

Caregiver's Organizer

Current medications:

Allergies:

Insurance Policy # / Group #:

Pediatrician:	Address
Phone	Fax/Email

Ear/Nose/Throat surgeon:	Address
Phone	Fax/Email

Surgical site:	Address
Phone	Fax/Email
Contact person	

Pharmacy:	Address
Phone	Fax/Email

Date of tour/visit to surgical center:	
Date of pre-operation testing:	
Date of surgical clearance exam at pediatrician:	
DATE of SURGERY:	
Post-surgical exam (with Surgeon)	
Post-surgical exam (with Pediatrician)	

Favorite ice cream flavors:

Appendix A – Timeline Review

When	What to Do
4-8 weeks before surgery	Introduce the information to your child and no, it is not too early to plant the seed.
3-4 weeks before surgery	Give your child more information. Read a book to your child about the procedure.
2-3 weeks before surgery	Give specific information to your child about his ENT doctor and upcoming experience.
1-2 weeks before surgery	Take your child shopping for postoperative food, treats, games and necessities. Visit the surgical site to acquaint your child with the place she will be going.
3-7 days before surgery	Get lab work done. Go to the library to borrow books and videos to entertain your child after surgery. Assemble a stash of quiet toys in one location in your home. Make an audio recording when you read to your child.
1-2 days before surgery	Bring your child to the pediatrician for surgical clearance. Fill all medications.
The Big Day!	Take your pre-packed bag. Wake your child up, get dressed, and go! Appear calm in front of your child.
During surgery	Grab something to eat and make your phone calls. Get things out of the way so you can be available to your child an hour later when he moves to the Recovery Room
After surgery	Once you are given the go ahead, sit with your child. Be patient and responsive to her cues. Give her your full attention. Follow instructions from medical staff.
At home	Make a medication chart to keep track of doses.
1 week after surgery	Return to the ENT for a check-up.
2 weeks after surgery	Return to normal. Return to school

Appendix B - What about Complications?

While complications following surgery are rare, it necessary for parents to be familiar with possible issues that would require immediate medical attention. If your child has other pre-existing medical issues or seizures, then she needs more intensive monitoring. This section of the book is intended only for you to read in advance of the surgery so you can be knowledgeable and prepared; it is not meant to scare you or to be shared with your child. Post-surgical complications may sound alarming but thankfully, are indeed rare.

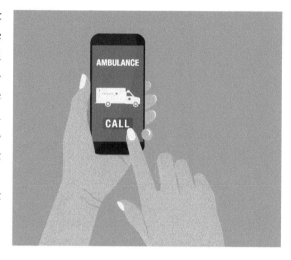

Bleeding

Bleeding can occur during surgery or afterward. Less than two percent of patients experience bleeding within the first 24 hours and less than three percent of patients have bleeding 5-10 days later when the child is home and scabs may separate from the surgical site, possibly reflecting an underlying infection or dehydration. Fewer bleeding complications are seen in younger children than teenagers, as their blood vessels are smaller. Should bleeding occur, however, you may be advised to give your child ice water to swallow or rinse with. If bleeding continues and is severe (more than two tablespoons of fresh blood), you will be among the 7-13 percent of families who will have to go to the Emergency Department, since intravenous fluids or a return to the operating room may be required (Messner, 2018). Although rare, bleeding may not be detectable because the child may be swallowing blood rather than spitting it out, which would result in abdominal pain, pallor, persistent vomiting and weakness after the child has already begun to feel better. Seldom is a transfusion needed for blood loss, but some families consider having designated donor directed blood available in advance of the procedure. Pain, persistent nausea or vomiting and dehydration are other reasons for follow up at the Emergency Department.

Infection

Infection may be signaled by prolonged pain or delayed healing. If fever rises (above 102 degrees Fahrenheit/38.9 Centigrade) or if an earache or fever of 101 degrees lasts for more than three days, you need to consult your physician.

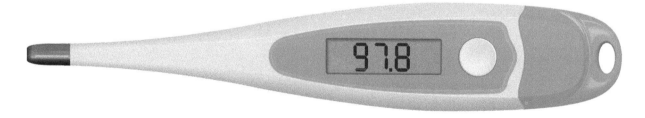

Anesthesia reactions

Children may be irritable and nauseous. Vomiting is not uncommon.

Dehydration

If your child does not take in enough liquids because of pain that causes difficulty swallowing, fluids may have to be supplied intravenously in the hospital. Signs of dehydration include dry mouth, refusal to drink for a 24 hour period, crying without tears, fatigue, weakness, dizziness or lightheadedness, decreased urination and/or thirst. Remember that drinking is much more important than eating! Difficulty breathing may be the result of extreme swelling of the area around the surgical site.

Other less worrisome consequences of adenotonsillectomies include bad breath during the healing process, changes in the sound of your child's speech, and weight gain due to improved health and eating habits. Pain is to be expected, and is often reported in the throat, ears and neck.

If your child is among the few who require a second surgical procedure due to complications, you can offer an explanation something to this effect:

> Do you remember how I (used to) tie your sneakers for you to keep them closed but sometimes they open again? Dr. ENT took out your tonsils already and closed up the place where your tonsils used to be. But since you just spat out some blood, the doctor said that it wasn't closed tight enough, so she needs to fix it a little more so that a lot of blood can't come out anymore. That means that you will go back to the special room for just a few more minutes, and go to sleep again so she can fix it and everything will stay just where it's supposed to be. Mommy and Daddy will stay with you, just like before."

But remember, complications are uncommon and can be addressed.

~ ~ ~

It is our sincerest hope that this book has supplied you with the information you will need to successfully support your child through a surgical experience. I hope that you will also read my other books:

Please Explain Anxiety to Me: Simple Biology and Solutions for Children and Parents

Please Explain Terrorism to Me: A Story for Children, P-E-A-R-L-S of Wisdom for their Parents
and our newest book,

Please Explain Time Out to Me: A Story for Children and Do-It-Yourself Manual for Parents.

References:

American Academy of Otolaryngology- Head and Neck Surgery. (2011). *Fact Sheet: Tonsillitis*, Patient Health Information. Alexandria, VA.

Baugh R. F., Archer S. M., Mitchell R. B., et al. (2017) Clinical practice guideline: Tonsillectomy in children. *Otolaryngol Head Neck Surg.*;144(1 Suppl):S1-30. doi: 10.1177/0194599810389949. PubMed PMID: 21493257 Retrieved from https://www.ncbi.nlm.nih.gov/pubmed/21493257

Garetz, S. L. (2018). Adenotonsillectomy for obstructive sleep apnea in children. Retrieved November 3, 2018, from https://www.uptodate.com/contents/adenotonsillectomy-for-obstructive-sleep-apnea-in-children

Hall MJ, Schwartzman A, Zhang J, Liu X. (2017) Ambulatory Surgery Data From Hospitals and Ambulatory Surgery Centers: United States, 2010. *Natl Health Stat Report. 2017 Feb;(102):1-15.* PubMed PMID: 28256998. Retrieved from: https://www.ncbi.nlm.nih.gov/pubmed/28256998

Messner, A. (2018). Tonsillectomy (with or without adenoidectomy) in children: Postoperative care and complications. Retrieved from https://www.uptodate.com/contents/tonsillectomy-with-or-without-adenoidectomy-in-children-postoperative-care-and-complications?topicRef=6296&source=see_link

Paradise, J., & Wald, E. (2018). Tonsillectomy and/or adenoidectomy in children: Indications and contraindications. Retrieved from https://www.uptodate.com/contents/tonsillectomy-and-or-adenoidectomy-in-children-indications-and-contraindications

Rowa, K., Antony, M., and Swinson, R. (2007) *Exposure and response prevention in psychological treatment of obsessive compulsive disorder: Fundamentals and beyond,* edited by MM Antony, C. Purdon and L.J. Summerfeldt published by American Psychological Association. pp 79-109.

Walton J, Ebner Y, Stewart MG, April MM. (2012) Systematic review of randomized controlled trials comparing intracapsular tonsillectomy with total tonsillectomy in a pediatric population. *Arch Otolaryngol Head Neck Surg.*;138(3):243-9. doi: 10.1001/archoto.2012.16. Review. PubMed PMID: 22431869. Retrieved from https://www.ncbi.nlm.nih.gov/pubmed/22431869

For further reading: Children's books and videos

Branford, A. (2011). *Violet Mackerel's remarkable recovery*. New York: Simon & Schuster.

Davison, M. (1992). *Rita Goes to the Hospital*. USA: Random House, Inc.

Densley, T and Palmer, N. (2016). *Hospital Adventures, Ollie's Tonsils*. USA: beanz books.

Hatkoff, J., Hatkoff, C., & Mets, M. (2004). *Good-bye tonsils!* New York: Puffin Books.

Hautzig, D. (1985). *A Visit to the Sesame Street Hospital*. New York: Random House/Children's Television Network.

Scarry, R. (1995). *The busy world of Richard Scarry: A big operation*. New York: Aladdin..

Tiny Docs (Director). (2016). *Shiver Me Tonsils* [Video file]. Retrieved November 3, 2018, from https://www.youtube.com/watch?v=YhvHUosBDto Produced by Tiny Docs.

About the Authors

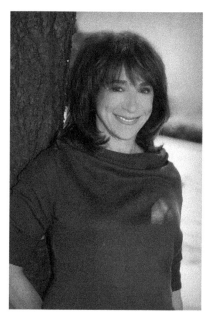

Dr. Laurie Zelinger, a Board Certified Psychologist, was born and raised in New York, and is a successful product of the New York City public school system. She earned her Master's degree and Professional Diploma from Queens College over 40 years ago and later went on to earn a Doctoral degree from Hofstra University. Dr. Laurie has held elected positions on the Board of Directors of the New York State Association for Play Therapy, and at the national level, she served on the prestigious American Board of Professional Psychology for two years. Her interest in children dates back to her days as a babysitter and became the foundation of her later pursuit of school psychology and play therapy. During the course of her professional career, Dr. Laurie Zelinger and her psychologist husband, Dr. Fred Zelinger, raised four sons. As parents, they learned firsthand the difference between reading about children and living with them.

This book represents the author's actual experience with her son Jordan's tonsillectomy and adenoidectomy, as well as her hope that others will benefit from this information. Her concept of preparing a child for surgery is based upon the premise that information and preparation will reduce anxiety and help families to better manage the experience. The suggested time lines may also be used as a guide for children undergoing other hospital procedures.

Dr. Laurie's ongoing devotion to children continues beyond her retirement as a school psychologist in the public school system, as she is now in full time private practice as a child psychologist and credentialed play therapist. She works and lives on Long Island, New York with her husband, Fred.

Dr. Perry Zelinger, the youngest of the Zelinger sons, is completing his Medical Residency in the Rusk Rehabilitation/ NYU Langone Health System. When time permits he enjoys an active lifestyle that includes soccer, surfing, bicycling and trivia games. Perry and his wife live with their two rescue dogs in Manhattan, New York.

We wish you a fast and easy recovery! Keep drinking fluids!
Dr. Laurie Zelinger and Dr. Perry Zelinger

Visit me at www.DrZelinger.com

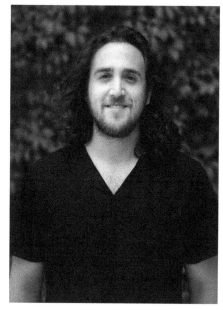

Please Explain Anxiety to Me

This book translates anxiety from the jargon of psychology into concrete experiences that children can relate to. Children and their parents will understand the biological and emotional components of anxiety responsible for the upsetting symptoms they experience. *Please Explain Anxiety to Me, 2nd Edition* gives accurate physiological information in child friendly language. A colorful dinosaur story explains the link between brain and body functioning, followed by practical therapeutic techniques that children can use to help themselves. Children will:

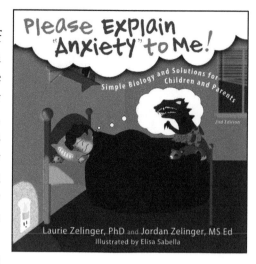

- learn that they can handle most issues if they are explained at their developmental level

- understand the brain/body connection underlying anxiety

- identify with the examples given

- find comfort and reassurance in knowing that others have the same experience

- be provided with strategies and ideas to help them change their anxiety responses

- be able to enjoy childhood and to give up unnecessary worrying

Therapists and Educators Praise "Please Explain Anxiety To Me, Second Edition"

"On any given day, around thirty percent of my patients have anxiety related symptoms. The simplicity and completeness of the explanations and treatment of anxiety given in this book is remarkable. Defining the cause, treating the core symptoms, and most importantly bringing it to a child's level accompanied by wonderful illustrations, is an incredible feat. I will definitely use this book in my practice."

Zev Ash, M.D. F.A.A.P., Pediatrician

"Anxiety is, of course, a complicated neuro-physiological process but it has been reduced to understandable terms in this brilliantly illustrated book for children. I would go even further and say that there are adults who could benefit from the straightforward approach."

Rick Ritter, MSW, author of *Coping with Physical Loss and Disability*

"This excellent book is perfect for parents to read and discuss with their children. It's also perfect for school professionals to use in the school setting."

Herb R. Brown, Ed.D., Superintendent of Schools Oceanside Public Schools, New York

"...A charming--and calming--explanation of anxiety that will help both children and their parents turn their internal worry switches to the OFF position."

Ellen Singer, New York Times-acclaimed bestselling author

Learn more at **www.DrZelinger.com**

ISBN 978-1-61599-216-4

From Loving Healing Press

Please Explain "Terrorism" to Me!
A Story for Children, P-E-A-R-L-S of Wisdom for their Parents

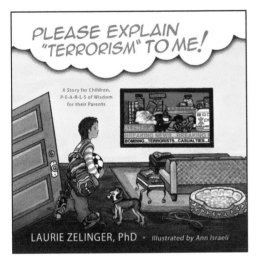

Complemented by exquisite, colorful artwork, Dr. Zelinger skillfully crafts an easily relatable children's story using everyday situations, around the oppressive concept of Terrorism in the news. With masterful understanding of the child's world, new and frightening concepts are introduced carefully and gently, with the child's perspective in mind.

Dr. Zelinger provides parent coaching to further the dialogue in her P-E-A-R-L-S of Wisdom section (Prepare, Explain, Answer, Reassure, Listen, Safeguard) where caregivers are given scripts to guide them, as well room for individuality. This pioneer book helps children and parents face a critical, often avoided topic with reassurance and calm.

"This book provides the 'PEARLS' of wisdom for parents and children to discuss a scary topic like terrorism in ways that promote healthy and authentic parent-child conversations that yield to mutual respect and bonding."
　　　　　—Marc A. Brackett, PhD., Director, Yale Center for Emotional Intelligence

"This fascinating guide amounts to a riveting lesson of clarity and to a masterpiece in bridging the unbridgeable."
　　　　　—Hon. Yehuda Lancry, Former Ambassador of Israel to the U.N.

"Dr. Zelinger uses common sense, a simple clarification of the basic issues, and reassurance to provide a deeper understanding of terrorism for kids—without a corresponding rise in anxiety."
　　　　　—Tomas W. Phelan, Ph.D., Psychologist/Author

Dr. Laurie Zelinger is a distinguished Board Certified Psychologist with Diplomate status in school psychology as well as a credentialed play therapist who serves on executive boards of state and national organizations. Ann Israeli is a retired art teacher, wall paper and textile designer.

Learn more at **www.DrZelinger.com**

ISBN 978-1-61599-291-1

From Loving Healing Press

Printed in the USA
CPSIA information can be obtained
at www.ICGtesting.com
LVHW062354080324
773808LV00015B/164